GUIDELINES FOR PROTECTING CONFIDENTIAL STUDENT HEALTH INFORMATION

National Task Force on Confidential Student Health Information

A Project of
American School Health Association
in Collaboration with
National Association of School Nurses
National Association of State School Nurse Consultants

Guidelines for Protecting Confidential Student Health Information

National Task Force on Confidential Student Health Information

Published by:
American School Health Association
7263 State Route 43 / P.O. Box 708
Kent, OH 44240

ISBN# 0-917160-00-2

For information, contact:
American School Health Association,
7263 State Route 43 / P.O. Box 708, Kent, OH 44240.

National Task Force
on Confidential Student Health Information

James F. Bogden, MPH
National Association of State Boards of Education

Elaine Brainerd, RN, MA, CSN
National Center for School Health Nursing

Judith Brotman
School Social Work Association of America

Charlotte Burt, RNC, MA
Chair
American School Health Association

John DiCecco, MSW
National Association of Social Workers

Kevin Dwyer
National Association of School Psychologists

Kate Fothergill
National Assembly on School-Based Health Care

Nora Howley
Council of Chief State School Officers

Mary Hughes Boyce Gelfman, MA, JD

Naomi Gittins, JD
National School Boards Association

Brenda Z. Greene
National School Boards Association

Ruth Ellen Luehr, MS, RN
Co-Chair 1997-98
National Association of State School Nurse Consultants

Phyllis Lewis, MSN, RN, FNP
Indiana Dept. of Education

National Task Force
on Confidential Student Health Information

Myrna Mandlawitz
National Association of State Directors of Special Education

Angela Oddone, MSW
American Psychological Association

Leslie J. Roberts II, MHA
American Association of School Administrators

Marcia Rubin, PhD, MPH
American School Health Association

Paul Sathrum
National Education Association

Nadine Schwab, BSN, MPH, PNP
Co-Chair, 1998-99
National Association of State School Nurse Consultants

Liane Summerfield, PhD
American Association of Colleges for Teacher Education

Susanne Tropez-Sims, MD
American Academy of Pediatrics

Elizabeth Truly, JD
American Federation of Teachers

Gwen Tucker
National Parent Teacher Association

Donna Zaiger, RN, BSN, CSN
Co-Chair
National Association of School Nurses

TABLE OF CONTENTS

PREFACE

The increasing presence in our nation's schools of students with chronic physical and emotional conditions, as well as behavioral or learning disorders, has made it more important than ever that school health professionals and administrators know how to handle confidential student health information. The right to confidentiality that these students and their families should expect is often challenged by their frequent need for a multitude of health services and special academic considerations that require physicians, school nurses, other pupil service specialists, teachers, aides, and parents to collaborate. Unfortunately, determining when and how confidential information about students should be shared without compromising their privacy is not straightforward. Several major problems often make it difficult to resolve this issue:

- *Conflicts between the policies, practices and administrative directives of local schools, legal obligations, and ethical standards of practice of school health professionals.*

For example, school health professionals might believe they should not divulge confidential information about a student to teachers or school administrators who believe they should have the information. This can result in tension and resentment.

- *Inconsistencies between federal and state laws addressing health and education.*

In most states, minors have the right to seek medical treatment without parental notification for specific conditions, such as HIV infection or AIDS, other sexually transmitted diseases, and drug or alcohol problems. These laws are based on the concern that minors might not seek treatment for these conditions if the information is not kept strictly confidential. In contrast, the federal Family Education Rights and Privacy Act (FERPA) which gives parents the right to access all their children's educational records, including their health records, does not make exception for these conditions.

• *Insufficient guidelines, policies, and procedures on
student health information.*
FERPA does not distinguish the special nature of
student health records and no national guidelines are
currently available that bring together the provisions
of FERPA, other relevant federal and state laws, and
ethical standards of health practice.

• *Inadequate pre-service and in-service preparation of
school personnel.*
Students' rights to confidentiality are often compromised by school staff who are not knowledgeable on the
subject of confidentiality. It is critical to ensure that all
school staff understand and adhere to appropriate principles and practices to protect confidentiality.

• *Communication difficulties.*
Parents, school staff, and health and educational
professionals often choose different words to express
similar ideas, or they might ascribe different mean-
ings to the same words, sometimes creating misun-
derstanding. Appendix A contains definitions of com-
monly used terms in this document. Furthermore, discussion about students often focuses on medical or
clinical diagnoses rather than their functional abilities and limitations which frequently leads to situations in which the students' privacy is violated.

To address these concerns, the American School
Health Association (ASHA), with funding support
from a cooperative agreement with the Division of
Adolescent and School Health (DASH) of the U.S.
Centers for Disease Control and Prevention (CDC),
convened the National Task Force on Confidential
Student Health Information to develop guidelines
that could assist school administrators, health professionals, and educators in developing appropriate policies and procedures that ensure that confidential student health information is appropriately protected.
Along with ASHA, the National Association of State
School Nurse Consultants (NASSNC) and the
National Association of School Nurses (NASN) co-
chaired the task force, which included representatives
from 20 national organizations or professional associ-
ations involved with children and school health. The
task force's charge was to identify practical guidelines

that would protect students confidentiality while 1) enabling health and mental health professionals to provide quality and continuous student services and 2) providing teachers and other school personnel with the health information they need to help students achieve their educational goals and maintain their health and safety. These guidelines are intended to help school personnel make thoughtful and appropriate decisions regarding disclosure or nondisclosure of student health information.

Mary H.B. Gelfman, MA, JD, drafted the first version of the document, which was edited by Marcia Rubin and members of the task force. A draft version circulated nationally for six months and was reviewed by numerous individuals representing various perspectives (Appendix B). Comments and suggestions were synthesized by Marcia Rubin and reviewed by the task force with significant contributions from Mary Gelfman, Nadine Schwab, and Elizabeth Truly. Susan Wooley, executive director of ASHA, contributed to the document continuously throughout the process and Judy Rollins, an editor for Pediatric Nursing reviewed the final version. The National Task Force is grateful for the prior deliberations and draft guidelines shared by the Connecticut Committee on the Confidentiality of Student Health Information (1994-96).

INTRODUCTION

What is *confidential student health information?* Briefly defined, it is personal, sensitive information obtained most often by a health professional concerning the physical, developmental, or mental health of an individual student. A student's health history might also include sensitive family information. "Confidentiality" is the implicit expectation that such information will not be communicated to a third party without explicit permission.[1] Since the National Task Force began its work in 1997, both the U.S. Congress and many state legislatures have considered the issue of confidentiality of health information. Congress has not yet passed a "Patients' Bill of Rights" protecting personal health information from inappropriate disclosure, but Maine and Massachusetts and several other states have amended their state medical records laws to extend these protections. Many other states are discussing similar changes.

Confidential information should not be confused with "privileged" communication. In many types of judicial proceedings, information received in confidence from a patient (or parent if the patient is a minor) by a physician or psychologist (and occasionally other health professionals) is protected from disclosure. Privilege laws vary by state.

Student health information can be oral, written, or transmitted electronically. Ensuring the confidentiality of this information is especially difficult because several school health professionals record this information in many locations in the school building or district. These might include physicians, nurse practitioners and school nurses, clinical psychologists, occupational and physical therapists, speech and language therapists, and school social workers.

At a minimum, school health records include information required by state law such as the following:

1) mandated immunizations;

2) health and physical assessment data;

3) health screenings for vision, hearing, scoliosis or cholesterol;

4) injury reports;

5) incident reports of alcohol or drug use in school;

6) health assessments and other evaluation reports related to eligibility for services under the Individuals with Disabilities Act (IDEA[2]) and §504 of the Rehabilitation Act of 1973;[3] and

7) referrals for suspected child abuse.

Additional health information might include:

- *records of student-initiated visits to the school health office, including assessments, interventions, and referrals (sometimes called process or narrative notes);*

- *records of meetings between education and health professionals for planning or identifying assessment measures, recommended interventions, and student outcomes;*

- *records for in-school medication, including original, signed orders from a physician, written consent from parent, and/or guardian to administer a drug, and medication logs for both routine and as-needed (PRN) medications;*

- *physicians' orders, correspondence, evaluation reports, copies of treatment records, institutional or agency records, and discharge summaries from outside health care providers or hospitals that have been released by parents to assist in planning individualized school health care or programs;*

- *evaluation reports or specialized assessments such as neurologic tests;*

- *individualized emergency care plans for students with special health care needs, including routine and emergency interventions and methods for evaluating student outcomes;*

- *health-related goals and objectives or an Individualized Healthcare Plan or part of a student's Individualized Education Program (IEP) for students whose health conditions affect their educational needs;*

* *psychologists' or guidance counselors' records of psychological test results, student interviews and counseling, consultations with school staff or parents, and referrals and consultation with outside counselors, therapists, psychologists or psychiatrists, all of which might be considered "mental health" records;*

* *school social workers' case histories, counseling notes and interviews, or their records of consultations with school staff, parents, outside counselors, therapists, psychologists, or psychiatrists; and*

* *case notes, evaluations, and interventions by other pupil services personnel.*

Access to health information varies by type and purpose. For example, IEPs might include some health information and they must be accessible to every member of the school staff responsible for implementing the IEP including administrators, supervisors, teachers, related service providers, and other school personnel such as paraprofessionals and assistants. Medical records from outside health care providers and hospitals, however, are generally accessible only to health professionals. Unfortunately, school staff often fail to distinguish different types of health information or recognize important privacy issues. They might not know, for example, that a doctor's explanation of why an immunization was not administered should not be included in the educational file; the physician's note might reveal sensitive information about the student such as a compromised immune system. Clearly, staff who provide health and education services to students must be adequately informed about a student's condition as the consequences of inadequate knowledge can be serious. The challenge is to establish a systematic structure for assuring appropriate safeguards to protect confidentiality while providing a mechanism that enables education and health professionals to share information that promotes the student's health and academic success.

*Guidelines for Protecting Confidential
Student Health Information* includes information
and guidance to address this important challenge.
Section I, Protecting Confidential Student Health
Information, reviews ethical responsibilities, legal
obligations, universal guidelines to protect confidentiality, and the role of parents in developing policies
and procedures. Section II, National Task Force
Recommendations and Guidelines, presents guidelines that local school districts can use when developing policies and practices.

PROTECTING CONFIDENTIAL STUDENT HEALTH INFORMATION

Students and their families have a right to expect that student health information, except in a few special cases, will be kept confidential and that only information necessary to provide appropriate health and educational services will be shared. Several issues must be considered when developing policies and procedures to protect and support this right.

Ethical Responsibilities

Four ethical issues linked to confidential information require thoughtful consideration and clear guidelines. These concern issues of privacy, the dictum "Do no harm," required disclosure for certain types of information, and the duty to warn.

Responsibility to Respect Privacy

"Privacy" is a fundamental right of individuals to be free from intrusion.[4] This right includes the expectation that confidential information will not be disclosed to third parties without explicit permission.[1,5] Professional educators are bound by the Code of Ethics from the National Education Association[6] which stipulates that the educator "shall not disclose information about students obtained in the course of professional service unless disclosure serves a compelling purpose or is required by law."

From the earliest days of the healing professions, health care providers recognized that patients are more likely to disclose all relevant information necessary for proper diagnosis and treatment if they know that private facts will be held in confidence.[7,8] By culture and tradition, people expect that health professionals will respect their privacy and that personal disclosures to health professionals will be kept confi-

---

Figure 1-1
Confidentiality Provisions from Codes of Professional Ethics

The School Nurse...	The Occupational Therapist...	The Speech & Hearing Therapist...
Provides health services, while recognizing each individual's inherent right to be treated with dignity and confidentiality...	Shall respect the confidential nature of information gained in any occupational therapy interaction...	Shall not reveal, without authorization, any professional or personal information about the person served professionally, unless doing so is necessary to protect the welfare of the person or the community.
Safeguards the client's right through confidentiality.	Shall take all due precautions to maintain the confidentiality of all verbal, written and electronic communications that are confidential.	
NASN	AOTA	ASHA

Exerpts from the Codes of Ethics of the National Association of School Nurses,
the American Occupational Therapy Association, and the American Speech and Hearing Association.

---

dential. Correspondingly, we recognize that violation of the patient/health professional relationship threatens effective health care. The special nature of the health care relationship has been confirmed and protected through the following:

- ethical codes of practice for all health professionals, regardless of their practice setting[9-11] (Figure 1-1);

- standards for health care institutions and agencies; and

- state laws and federal statutes and regulations regarding health assessments, treatment, counseling, and referral.[1]

Responsibility to Do No Harm

When contemplating a disclosure of confidential health information, school health professionals will want to review their professional practice standards and the relevant ethical issues while carefully considering the best interests of the individual student. Before making a decision several questions must be answered:[12]

- Can the truth of the information be confirmed?

- To what extent will disclosure limit the individual's freedom and autonomy?

- To what extent is the individual's or his/her family's privacy violated by disclosure?

- Can disclosure be justified for the student's benefit?
- To what extent might personal bias affect my judgment?
- Will a decision to disclose do less harm to the individual than not disclosing?
- Would disclosure jeopardize the fidelity of the health care relationship?[13-15]

Unfortunately, many of the confidentiality issues that arise concerning student health issues do not have simple answers. For example, many health professionals struggle with the issue of student confidences concerning sexual activity, birth control, abortion, pregnancy and sexually transmitted diseases, including HIV. These professionals are advised to consider the individual's competence or possible danger to others, refer to the laws and court decisions in their state, and review local district policies for guidance. At least one federal court has concluded that the Constitution does not require schools to notify a student's parents or the father about a pregnancy or about the student's plans for the pregnancy[16] but other federal or state courts might rule differently. As a general rule, only after serious and deliberate consideration, and then only when the balance clearly tips in favor of disclosure, should confidential information be shared.

Responsibility to Disclose Some Types of Information

In a few specific circumstances the responsibility to disclose information clearly outweighs individual claims for confidentiality.

Suspected Child Abuse

Both the federal Child Abuse Prevention and Treatment Act and state laws require individuals whose employment places them in contact with children (e.g., teachers and other school employees, physicians and nurses, child care workers) to report suspected child abuse, neglect, or imminent danger of abuse.[17] These "mandated reporters" can share confidential information with the appropriate designated authority to help assess and monitor the student's health in relation to suspected abuse and to intervene to protect the student.[1, 18-21]

School officials and health professionals often are concerned about where to keep the record of this report, which identifies both the student and the reporter, and whether parents have access to the report. In response to an inquiry, the Family Policy Compliance Office of the U.S. Department of Education concluded that under the Family Education Rights and Privacy Act of 1974 (FERPA, the Buckley Amendment) the report of suspected child abuse was accessible to parents but that school administrators may copy the record to give to the parents and delete the name of the reporter from the copy.[22]

Self-Injury or Suicide

When a health care professional determines that a student is at serious risk of self-harm, the obligation to protect the individual supersedes privacy issues.[23]

Possible Harm to Another Person

If health professionals learn of a major threat to the health and safety of students, such as a planned homicide, gang violence, or rape, they have an obligation, recognized by FERPA and other laws as well as by ethical practice standards to intervene. These actions might necessitate the sharing of appropriate but confidential information to prevent significant and imminent harm.

Duty to Warn

When information is received in confidence by a physician or psychologist (and occasionally other health professionals as defined by state law), this information is protected from disclosure in many types of judicial proceedings. Just as there are limits to confidentiality in some circumstances, however, there are also limits to "privilege." The "duty to warn" evolved as a legal principle from a California case in which a college health service psychologist learned that one of his student patients intended to kill another student. The psychologist asked the campus police to detain the patient, but the police did so for only a short time. Later, the patient killed the student. The victim's parents sued the psychologist for failure to warn the victim. In his defense, the psychologist cited "privilege" and confidentiality as a limiting factor. The Court, however, held that a "duty to warn" a possible victim overrode confidentiality protections.[24] "We conclude that the professional code of ethics favoring protection of the confidential character of patient-psychotherapist communications must yield to the extent to which disclosure is essential to avert danger to others. The protective privilege ends where the public peril begins."[17, 24, 25] Since this ruling, there has been a trend to require psychiatrists and other providers in privileged relationships to take "reasonable steps" to protect an intended victim when they learn that a patient presents a "serious danger of violence" to a specific, identifiable person. These reasonable steps might not include revealing the name of the person threatening the crime unless a court order requires it.[26]

Legal Obligations

The ability of more students with various health problems to attend school has increased the amount of confidential health information with which schools must contend. In addition, these students often require individualized education programs (IEPs), special classroom accommodations, and a variety of support services.[27] School districts are bound by several state and federal laws affecting education and health practices in schools including (FERPA),[28] the Individuals with Disabilities Act (IDEA),[2] various rulings from the Office for Civil Rights of the U.S. Department of Education, and state laws regarding the medical treatment of minors, professional licensure, and medical records.

All professional staff working in schools should become familiar with relevant laws affecting student records. A helpful resource is *Protecting the Privacy of Student Records: Guidelines for Educational Agencies*[4] written by The Council of Chief State School Officers' (CCSSO). It includes detailed discussions of the various federal laws that protect student information; the responsibilities of school districts when collecting and storing this information; general practices for sharing confidential student information outside the student's school; and several useful model forms for local school district use. Unfortunately, the CCSSO report addresses student records in general; it does not discuss the special problems and issues concerning student health information. Several states, however, including Connecticut, Maryland, Massachusetts, Oregon, and Washington, have developed materials that address several health-related confidentiality issues.[1, 29-33] A few journal articles also have addressed student health records.[19, 34, 35]

The following discussion provides a brief introduction to and highlights certain aspects of key federal laws that schools should consider when developing policies and procedures to protect confidential student health information.

Family Educational Rights and Privacy Act of 1974 (FERPA)

FERPA or the Buckley Amendment[28] protects the privacy of students and their parents by restricting access to school records in which individual student information is kept. Only "school officials with legitimate education interest" can directly access students' records. The school district must define "legitimate education interest" and specify the criteria for deciding who has this interest. FERPA provides parents with access to all their child's school records, including health records, and stipulates that these records may not be released outside the school without specific parental consent except in a few circumstances:

• when a student intends to enroll in another school;

- research and/or evaluation studies focused on improving instruction or care; or

- an emergency in which disclosure is necessary to protect the health or safety of the student or other individuals. Only that information necessary to reduce the danger may be shared and then only with necessary medical, administrative or law enforcement personnel.

Because of increasing concerns about violence and school safety, the Office of Juvenile Justice and Delinquency Prevention in the U.S. Department of Justice and the U.S. Department of Education's Family Policy Compliance Office have clarified FERPA consent exceptions related to juvenile justice issues.[36] In their 1997 publication, *Sharing Information*, they state that in cases of violent or abusive behavior, the following information can be disclosed without parental consent:

- communication between mandated reporters and a child protection agency concerning a student who might be a victim of abuse (the Child Abuse Protection Act provides additional information); and

- information that enables the juvenile justice system to "effectively serve" a student prior to adjudication in states where laws allow for this.

FERPA requires school districts to inform parents in writing, every year, of the district's policies and administrative procedures regarding student records; frequently this annual notice is summarized in student handbooks or similar documents. Parents should also receive information on the additional protections afforded student health information, the types of school-based or school-linked health services available to students, and the names and phone numbers of the school's health professionals. In addition the parental notice should explain in clear, easily understood language (in translation, if necessary) the rights of parents and of young people, the limits of confidentiality, and relevant concepts such as "informed consent." The U.S. Department of Education (USDoEd) has produced a model notice of parents' rights under FERPA and a model school district records policy, outlining these protections (Appendix C). The Family Policy Compliance Office of USDoEd Phone: 202/260-3887 can provide clarification and technical assistance about the FERPA regulations.

Protection of Pupil Rights Amendment

In addition to FERPA, school districts that receive funding from USDoED are subject to the Protection of Pupil Rights Amendment, the Hatch Amendment.[37] This amendment requires state education agencies, local school districts, and USDoED contractors to obtain the prior consent of a student's parent or guardian (or the student if an adult or an emancipated minor) before students complete a survey **if** all four of the following conditions pertain: 1) USDoED funds were used to develop or implement the survey; 2) the survey is administered in an elementary or secondary school; 3) the student is *required* to complete the survey; and 4) the survey asks the student to reveal information about any of the following:

- political affiliation;

- psychological problems potentially embarrassing to the student or his/her family;

- sexual behavior and attitudes;

- illegal, anti-social, self-incriminating, or demeaning behavior;

- critical appraisal of family members;

- privileged relationships, such as with a physician or minister; and

- income (other than that required by law to determine eligibility for participation in a school program or for receiving financial assistance).

Similar information may be collected without parental consent by school health professionals during routine health assessments or counseling or by school programs funded through other sources.

Individuals with Disabilities Education Act (IDEA)

IDEA requires considerations beyond those of FERPA: (a) parent notification concerning the purposes of collected student information; (b) procedures for storing, retaining, and destroying records; (c) training for all staff members who collect or use information related to special education students; and (d) publication of names and positions of staff members with access to student information. Parents of a student eligible for special education may designate a representative to review their child's records (34 C.F.R. 300.560 - 300.577).

When students with disabilities misbehave in school, school health professionals sometimes become involved in determining whether the misbehavior is related to the student's disability or medication (manifestation determination). Section 615(k)(9) of IDEA states that (a) a school is not prohibited from reporting a crime committed by a child with a disability to appropriate authorities, and (b) if a school does report a crime, copies of the special education and disciplinary records of the student are to be provided for consideration by appropriate authorities to whom it reports the crime. School health professionals should take steps to ensure that confidential health information irrelevant to the crime is not released inappropriately.

State Laws Concerning Minors' Rights to Consent to Medical Treatment

In every state, "mature minors" may obtain medical and mental health treatment for certain conditions e.g., substance abuse or sexually transmitted diseases, without parental consent. [8, 13, 38-41] (Table 1) States have identified different ages for defining a "mature minor," i.e., one who can understand his or her situation, the treatment options available and the potential positive and negative outcomes of each option. "Emancipated minors" are those individuals younger than 18 who are married, supporting themselves, or living independently.

Table 1 - Confidential Care for Minors *Reproduced with the permission of the Alan Guttmacher Institute from: Teenagers' right to consent to reproductive health care, Issues in Brief, The Alan Guttmacher Institute: New York and Washington, 1997*

State	Contraceptive Services	Prenatal Care	STD-HIV/AIDS Services	Treatment for Alcohol and/or Drug Abuse	Outpatient Mental Health Services	General Medical Care	Abortion Services[1]
Alabama	NL	MC	MC[2,3,4]	MC	MC	MC[5]	PC
Alaska	MC	MC	MC	NL	NL	MC[6]	NL
Arizona	NL	NL	MC	MC[2]	NL	NL	NL
Arkansas	MC	MC[7]	MC	NL	NL	MC[8]	PN[9]
California	MC	MC[7]	MC[2,10]	MC[2,4]	MC[2]	NL	NL
Colorado	MC	NL	MC[10]	MC	MC[4,11]	NL	NL
Connecticut	NL	NL	MC[10]	MC	MC	NL	MC
Delaware	MC[2,4]	MC[2,4,7,8]	MC[2,4,10]	MC[2]	NL	NL	PN[12]
Dist. Columbia	MC	MC[8]	MC	MC	MC	NL	MC
Florida	MC[13]	MC[8]	MC[3]	MC	MC[14]	NL	NL
Georgia	MC	MC[7]	MC[3,4]	MC[4]	NL	NL	PN
Hawaii	MC[4,15]	MC[4,7,15]	MC[4,15]	MC[4]	NL	NL	NL
Idaho	MC	NL	MC[3,15]	MC	NL	MC	PN[9,16]
Illinois	MC[13]	MC[8]	MC[2,3]	MC[2]	MC[2,4]	MC[6,8,17]	NL
Indiana	NL	NL	MC	MC	NL	NL	PC
Iowa	NL	NL	MC[10,18]	MC	NL	NL	PN[12]
Kansas	NL	MC[8,19]	MC[4]	MC	NL	MC[8,19,20]	PN
Kentucky	MC[4]	MC[4,7]	MC[3,4]	MC[4]	MC[4,20]	MC[4,6,8]	PC
Louisiana	NL	NL	MC[4]	MC[4]	NL	MC[4,8]	PC
Maine	MC[13]	NL	MC[4]	MC	MC[4]	NL	MC[21]

MC = Minor authorized to consent or decide. **PC** = Parental consent explicitly required. **PN** = Parental notice explicitly required. **NL** = No law found

Table 1 - Confidential Care for Minors (Continued) *Reproduced with the permission of the Alan Guttmacher Institute from: Teenagers' right to consent to reproductive health care, Issues in Brief, The Alan Guttmacher Institute: New York and Washington, 1997*

State	Contraceptive Services	Prenatal Care	STD-HIV/AIDS Services	Treatment for Alcohol and/or Drug Abuse	Outpatient Mental Health Services	General Medical Care	Abortion Services[1]
Maryland	MC[4]	MC[4]	MC[4]	MC[4]	MC[4,20]	MC[4,6]	PN[22]
Massachusetts	NL	MC[7]	MC	MC[2]	MC[20]	MC[6,8,17]	PC
Michigan	NL	MC[4]	MC[4,10]	MC[4]	MC[15]	NL	PC
Minnesota	NL	MC[4]	MC[4]	MC[4]	NL	MC[6]	PN[9]
Mississippi	MC	MC[8]	MC[3]	MC[4,11]	NL[23]	MC[23]	PC[9]
Missouri	NL	MC[4,7,8]	MC[4,8]	MC[4,8]	NL	MC[6,8]	PC
Montana	MC[4]	MC[4,8]	MC[4,8,10]	MC[4,8]	MC[20]	MC[4,6,8]	PN
Nebraska	NL	NL	MC	MC	NL	NL	PN
Nevada	NL	NL	MC[3]	MC	NL	MC	NL
New Hampshire	NL	NL	MC[15]	MC[2]	NL	MC	NL
New Jersey	NL	MC[4,8]	MC[4,8]	MC[4]	NL	MC[4,6,8,17]	NL
New Mexico	MC	NL	MC[10]	MC	MC	NL	NL
New York	MC	MC	MC[10]	MC	MC	MC[6]	NL
North Carolina	MC	MC[7]	MC[3]	MC	MC	NL	PC[12]
North Dakota	NL	NL	MC[15]	MC[15]	NL	NL	PC[9]
Ohio	NL	NL	MC[10]	MC	MC[15]	NL	PN[24]
Oklahoma	MC[4,25]	MC[4,7]	MC[3,4]	MC[4]	NL	MC[4,6,8]	NL
Oregon	MC[4]	NL	MC[3,8]	MC[4,15]	MC[15]	MC[4,8,11]	NL
Pennsylvania	NL	MC	MC[3]	MC[4]	NL	MC[25,26]	PC
Rhode Island	NL	NL	MC[10]	MC	NL	NL	PC

MC = Minor authorized to consent or decide. **PC** = Parental consent explicitly required. **PN** = Parental notice explicitly required. **NL** = No law found

Table 1 - Confidential Care for Minors (Continued) *Reproduced with the permission of the Alan Guttmacher Institute from: Teenagers' right to consent to reproductive health care, Issues in Brief, The Alan Guttmacher Institute: New York and Washington, 1997*

State	Contraceptive Services	Prenatal Care	STD-HIV/AIDS Services	Treatment for Alcohol and/or Drug Abuse	Outpatient Mental Health Services	General Medical Care	Abortion Services[1]
South Carolina	NL[27]	NL[27]	NL[27]	NL[27]	NL[27]	MC[27]	PC[12]
South Dakota	NL	NL	MC	MC	NL	NL	PN
Tennessee	MC	MC	MC[3]	MC	MC[20]	NL	NL
Texas	NL	MC[4,7,8]	MC[3,4,8]	MC[4]	MC	NL	NL
Utah	NL	MC	MC	NL	NL	NL	PN[9,16]
Vermont	NL	NL	MC[2,3]	MC[2]	NL	NL	NL
Virginia	MC	MC	MC[3]	MC	MC	NL	PN
Washington	NL	NL	MC[3,15]	MC[15]	MC[14]	NL	NL
West Virginia	NL	NL	MC	MC	NL	NL	PN[28]
Wisconsin	NL	NL	MC	MC[2]	NL	NL	PC[12]
Wyoming	MC	NL	MC[3]	NL	NL	NL	PC
Total MC	24	28	50	46	22	22	3
Total PC/PN	0	0	0	0	0	0	30
Total NL	27	23	1	5	29	29	18

MC = Minor authorized to consent or decide. **PC** = Parental consent explicitly required. **PN** = Parental notice explicitly required. **NL** = No law found

Table Notes

1. Includes only laws that are currently enforced. These laws include a judicial bypass except where indicated. Eight states (AK, AZ, CA, CO, IL, NV, NM, and TN) have parental consent or notice laws that have been enjoined and therefore are not in effect.
2. Minor must be 12 or older.
3. State officially classifies HIV/AIDS as an STD or infectious disease, for which minors may consent to testing and treatment.

Table Notes *(Continued)*

4. Doctor may notify parents.
5. Minor must be 14 or older, a high school graduate, married, pregnant or a parent.
6. Minor may consent if has a child.
7. Excludes abortion.
8. Includes surgery.
9. Involvement of both parents required in most cases.
10. Law explicitly authorizes minors to consent to HIV testing and/or treatment.
11. Minor must be 15 or older.
12. Notice or consent may be given to or by grandparent or, alternatively, in DE to a licensed mental health professional, or in WI by another adult relative over age 25.
13. Minor may consent if has a child or doctor believes minor would suffer "probable" health hazard if services not provided; in FL and IL, also if minor is pregnant; in IL, also if referred by doctor, clergyman or Planned Parenthood clinic.
14. Minor must be at least 13.
15. Minor must be at least 14.
16. Does not include judicial bypass.
17. Minor may consent if pregnant.
18. Parent must be notified if HIV test is positive.
19. Minor may consent if parent is not "available," or in the case of general medical care, "immediately available."
20. Minor must be 16 or older.
21. Minor may be counseled by physician or a counselor in lieu of obtaining parental consent or court authorization.
22. Law has no judicial bypass; however, a physician may waive notification if the minor does not live with a parent; or if doctor determines that the minor is mature enough to give informed consent or that notification may lead to physical or emotional abuse of the minor or otherwise to be contrary to her best interests; or if reasonable effort to give notice was unsuccessful.
23. Any minor who is mature enough to understand the nature and consequences of the proposed medical or surgical treatment may consent.
24. Stepparent, grandparent, or sibling over age 21 may be notified if minor files affidavit stating she fears physical, sexual or severe emotional abuse from parent.
25. Minor may consent if she has ever been pregnant.
26. Minor may consent if has graduated from high school.
27. Any minor 16 and older may consent to any health service other than operations. Health services may be rendered to minors of any age without parental consent when the provider believes services are necessary.
28. Notice or judicial bypass can be waived if second physician determines that minor is mature enough to give consent or that notice would not be in her best interest.

In some states, "emancipated minors" are considered adults. A federal law provides protection to minors seeking and receiving alcohol and drug abuse treatment. Federal regulations regarding the confidentiality of alcohol and drug abuse patient records (42 CFR Part 2) apply to assessment, diagnosis, counseling, group counseling, treatment, or referral for treatment in most programs in which students participate. They forbid the release of any information without a patient's consent, even if the patient is in school and under 18 years of age. Nonetheless, if referral or treatment information is documented in the school health record, it is subject to FERPA and parents can access the information.

In 1990, USDoED and the Substance Abuse and Mental Health Services Administration issued a joint opinion suggesting several potential solutions to this dilemma. None of the suggestions is wholly satisfactory, however, and school health professionals are advised to seek information about potential confidentiality conflicts from their state attorney general or the Family Compliance Office in the USDoED.

Universal Guidelines to Protect Confidentiality

Many issues are at stake when seeking to protect the privacy of students and respond to the obligations established by law. Districts that have clear rules, procedures, policies, standards, security, and sanctions can simultaneously protect and serve the best interests of students, their families, and the districts themselves.

Nowhere has this been more obvious than in cases involving HIV-infected students.[42,43] The most widely publicized case was that of Ryan White who was barred from high school after his mother mentioned to two teachers that he had AIDS. After winning a lengthy and very public court battle, Ryan and his family moved to another town where he entered high school without controversy. In another case, in December, 1985, the Longmeadow, Massachusetts superintendent of schools paved the way for a teenager with hemophilia and HIV infection to attend school while protecting the student's privacy and without a single student withdrawing from school. During this same period, the admission of an unnamed child with AIDS to a New York City school triggered a boycott by protesting parents in 63 other New York City schools. In still another case two years later, a Florida court upheld the right of three brothers with hemophilia and HIV infection to attend an elementary school.[44] After the family received death threats, the school offered workshops for parents. Ultimately, however, even the mayor withdrew his child from school and the family was forced into hiding and subsequently moved out of town.

What distinguished those schools that effectively managed the controversy surrounding school attendance by children with AIDS from those where controversy got out of hand?

1) Principals and superintendents provided factual information about HIV infection and AIDS to parents, students, and staff in a variety of ways including meetings and mailings, and established information hotlines to deal with rumors and misinformation.

2) Districts followed policy guidelines related to accommodating children with communicable diseases or disabilities. School administrators did not disclose the name, age, or gender of HIV-infected children.

3) Administrators educated themselves about HIV infection and AIDS and exhibited leadership and openness in dealing with students, staff, parents and the community. They answered the questions they could address and promptly referred other questions to experts. In addition, they invited rather than suppressed discussion.

In most court cases involving children with HIV infection who had either been barred from school or subjected to isolation, the courts have compelled schools to admit the child and provide educational services based on the child's needs. In many cases, the courts awarded parents the attorneys' fees as well. In decisions across the country,[45-47] courts have upheld school district and state department of education policies that provide confidentiality protection for students infected with HIV. *Someone at School has AIDS*, published by the National Association of State Boards of Education (NASBE), provides guidance for schools wishing to establish specific policies related to HIV infection and AIDS.[48] In addition to strict confidentiality standards, such policies should include procedures for dealing with situations where there is an exchange of blood or other bodily fluids (student-to-student or student-to-staff) and a mechanism for school staff to inform school health professionals of any situation where there has been such an exchange so that parents or physicians of the involved persons can be notified.

When districts have clear, thorough and consistent policies and procedures in place, school health professionals can work effectively with school administrators and teachers to serve the interests of all children and parents. Just as universal precautions and procedures protect everyone equally, the confidentiality principles that protect the privacy of HIV- infected children apply to protect the confidentiality of ALL student health information.

Parents As Partners

Parents must participate fully with health professionals, school administrators, teachers and support staff in the development of their district's policies and procedures. All families, not just those who regularly attend school meetings, should be actively recruited to participate when districts formulate guidelines that address confidential student health information. Sincere outreach strategies include translating communications from the school for non-English-speaking families and providing regularly scheduled and convenient opportunities for parents to talk with principals and other administrative staff. Professional development programs for teachers and administrators on enhancing their relationships with parents are also important. In January 1997, the National PTA[49] developed standards for bolstering parent involve-

Figure 1-2
National Parent Teacher Association
National Standards For Parent/Family Involvement

Standard I: Communicating - Communication between home and school is regular, two-way, and meaningful.

Standard II: Parenting - Parenting skills are promoted and supported.

Standard III: Student Learning - Parents play an integral role in assisting student learning.

Standard IV: Volunteering - Parents are welcome in the school, and their support and assistance are sought.

Standard V: School Decision Making and Advocacy - Parents are full partners in the decisions that affect children and families.

Standard VI: Collaborating with Community - Community resources are used to strengthen schools, families, and student learning.

ment in education (Figure 1-2). Parents who are well-informed and confident that the district respects their child's rights and privacy are more likely to become fully participating partners with school staff.

NATIONAL TASK FORCE RECOMMENDATIONS AND GUIDELINES

The National Task Force recommends that all school personnel regard as confidential all information related to a specific student's physical, mental, and developmental health status, whether that information is written, oral, or in electronic form. This information is subject to the protections required by federal and state law and the local school district's confidentiality policies and practices. School districts have a responsibility to ensure that a specific student's health information is maintained, stored, retrieved, and transferred in ways that protect students' and their family's privacy. This responsibility includes adopting specific policies, developing clear administrative procedures that protect confidential student health information, identifying sanctions and penalties when rules are violated, and providing staff training that addresses uniform implementation of the policies and procedures.[1,35]

Clear policies and procedures help school health professionals balance the need to protect confidentiality with the need to provide relevant information to other school personnel in order to provide students with appropriate educational programs and a safe environment. The following guidelines are intended to help school personnel make thoughtful and appropriate decisions regarding student health information and establish policies and procedures for ensuring that confidential student health information is appropriately protected.

Recommended Guidelines for Protecting Confidential Student Health Information

Guideline I

Distinguish student health information from other types of school records.

Guideline II

Extend to school health records the same protections granted medical records by federal and state law.

Guideline III

Establish uniform standards for collecting and recording student health information.

Guideline IV

Establish district policies and standard procedures for protecting confidentiality during the creation, storage, transfer, and destruction of student health records.

Guideline V

Require written, informed consent from the parent and, when appropriate, the student, to release medical and psychiatric diagnoses to other school personnel.

Guideline VI

Limit the disclosure of confidential health information within the school to information necessary to benefit students' health or education.

Guideline VII

Establish policies and standard procedures for requesting needed health information from outside sources and for releasing confidential health information, with parental consent, to outside agencies and individuals.

Guideline VIII

Provide regular, periodic training for all new school staff, contracted service providers, substitute teachers, and school volunteers concerning the district's policies and procedures for protecting confidentiality.

Guideline I

Distinguish student health information from other types of school records.

FERPA allows school district employees "with legitimate educational interest" to access student records without parental consent. FERPA requires a district to define who has "legitimate educational interest" in different types of school records and allows districts to establish special standards for access to certain types of records. With regard to school health records, it is recommended that school districts:

1) establish a classification system that recognizes health records as distinct from other educational records;

2) define "legitimate health interest;" and

3) identify specific criteria by which individuals are designated as "school officials with legitimate health interest" to directly access students' health records. Many school districts classify information about individual students in three categories:[19,50]

Class A: Academic information such as grade transcripts and attendance information and educational records, including IEPs for students with special education needs.

Class B: Temporary records that are usually discarded at the end of the school year or sooner.

Class C: Sensitive records, such as child abuse reports, nursing records, medical and psychiatric reports, hospital records, psychological test results, and counseling records.

Generally, only professionally prepared and licensed health care providers, such as physicians, nurses, social workers, psychologists, and occupational and physical therapists working in that capacity in the school district, should have access to Class C health records and then only if they are relevant to their discipline or practice. When teachers or others need information that might be contained in the Class C health record, the maker of the record or appropriately designated health professional with whom the maker regularly collaborates to directly serve the student should communicate that information, for example, through an emergency or daily health care plan.

In cases where a site lacks health professionals on a regular basis, the district should consult state law and discuss the issue with parents, the school board, and senior administration. In this case, some school districts allow the principal to access some Class C records, such as medication records, for use in a crisis.

Ideally, however, access should be strictly limited to licensed health professionals who originate the records because they can best interpret their meaning. If a decision is made to disclose sensitive information, the maker of the record or appropriately designated official should assume responsibility for communicating information necessary to benefit the health, safety, and educational progress of the student and for reminding the recipient to protect the information from further disclosure.

Guideline II

Extend to school health records the same protections granted medical records by federal and state law.

The U.S. Department of Education has ruled that medical records sent to schools are subject to FERPA regulations and thus must be accessible to parents, be kept confidential, and not be re-released without parental consent.[51, 52] Apart from allowing access to parents, however, medical records in the school health file remain protected under the state's laws regarding medical records, mental health records, or social service records.

School district policy should ensure that health records generated within the school by school health professionals are granted the same protections as medical records. Under such a policy, school health professionals may legally share appropriate health information with other school health professionals, those designated as having "legitimate health interest" within the district, and individuals providing direct school health and education services to students but restrict direct access to the record without written, informed consent from the student, or the parent if the student is under 18 years of age.

Guideline III

Establish uniform standards for collecting and recording student health information.

Clear procedures for collecting and recording health information help ensure quality care and provide accountability. Uniform and consistent documentation should include assessments, referrals, expected student outcomes, consultations, interventions, and evaluation data.[21] School health professionals within a district should discuss the documentation procedures they will follow. All methods of documentation should:

• promote optimal student health and learning;

• meet standards of professional practice and state law;

• provide necessary data for accountability; and

• contribute to timely and quality health care.[21]

Failure to appropriately conduct and contemporaneously document a health assessment exposes the health professional to liability if the student experiences an adverse outcome. For example, in a case involving a student with asthma who died a few hours after the second of two visits to a school nurse, the court required a review of the school health record and found that both the nurse's assessment of the student's condition and the record were inadequate.[53]

Personal Notes

Under FERPA, the "personal notes" of school health professionals' are not considered part of the school records only when they are primarily "memory joggers," are kept in the sole possession of the maker, and are not accessible or revealed, orally or otherwise, to any other person except a temporary substitute for the maker of the record. All information pertinent to appropriate care should be adequately documented in the record.

Guideline IV

Establish district policies and standard procedures for protecting confidentiality during the creation, storage, transfer, and destruction of student health records.

Given the increasing documentation required for a multitude of programs funded with federal and state monies, districts need specific policies on collecting, maintaining, storing, transferring, and destroying student health information. The state custodian of records, the state library, or the Secretary of State should be able to provide guidance on developing these policies, which must be consistent with state law.

Record Creation

Respect for student and family confidentiality is demonstrated when interviews with students, parents, or staff members concerning health information take place in private offices. When student health information is discussed over the telephone, calls should be made from private offices, not in the presence of other students or staff members. Discussion of confidential information related to a specific student should end whenever a third party enters the room. Records containing student health information should never be left open on top of a desk. Nor should confidential information be left as a message with a secretary, on voice mail or answering machines, or on an electronic mail system.[1,4] When records are being typed, entered into computer data bases, copied, or telecopied, they should be protected from casual observers by covers or screens. Copiers and fax machines should be located away from student and staff traffic.

Despite standards to the contrary, many schools still use a chronological tracking log to record visits to the health office. This procedure violates privacy because it lists the student's name and the reason for the visit where anyone can see it. Such a log also makes it difficult to track a particular student's visits. To protect privacy and insure quality of practice, individual student records should be used instead, e.g., 5" x 7" cards, individual pages in a notebook, or secure computer files.[18-21, 34]

Record Storage

Records might be stored in different places depending on the need for frequent access or the category of record. Regardless of where they are stored, student health information should be stored in locked file cabinets or secure computer files. FERPA requires that access records or logs be maintained, showing the name, title, date of access, and reason for access by individuals other than the maker of the record or those authorized to directly access the record. If information from the record is copied or released to third parties, the nature of the disclosure should be documented along with written parental consent for the disclosures.

During the next decade, vast amounts of confidential student information, including health information, will be stored in computer files. Available computer software can ease the burden of record keeping, allow retrieval of an individual student's health history, or aggregate school health statistics for reporting purposes.[54, 55] On the other hand, computerized records introduce new concerns about confidentiality protections. For the Record, a 1997 publication of the National Research Council,[5] suggests several steps for protecting electronic health information:

- require individual authentication of users to access files;

- limit access to only a few individuals;

- establish audit trails of who accessed specific files;

- place the computer in a secure area;

- develop a disaster, back-up recovery plan;

- limit and protect remote access points;

- do not link with external electronic communications; and

• perform routine system assessment.

Implementing these steps can make the security of electronic records similar to safeguards for paper records.

Transfer of Health Information

Most school districts transfer records to help ensure that schools can promptly and appropriately serve new students. FERPA does not require consent from a parent to send school records to another school where the student intends to enroll, but neither does it require school districts to transfer all records. School policies should include information on the district's procedures when school records are requested from another school to which the student intends to transfer. In the absence of such policies, FERPA requires schools to make a reasonable attempt to notify parents or eligible students when a request is received. Parents may request deletion of certain information before school records are sent.

Under some state laws, medical records released from a third party to a school may not be re-released or transferred without consent. Because school personnel are often unaware of the existence or implications of such state laws, school districts' policies should incorporate state law restrictions on re-disclosure. In addition, when transferring school health records, they should be labeled **CONFIDENTIAL** and mailed to the appropriate health professional by certified mail, which provides an acknowledgment of receipt.[1,5] Transmission by telefax should use a cover sheet addressed to a specific individual and should be clearly marked **CONFIDENTIAL**. Ideally, the recipient should be present to receive the fax.

Record Destruction

A school district should establish policies specifying which records to destroy at the end of each school year, which records to destroy when a student leaves a school, and how long to keep health records if a student leaves the district. Some state regulations provide state-wide retention and destruction schedules and the federal government currently requires maintaining records of federally-funded programs at least three years for audit purposes. Under FERPA, however, no records can be destroyed while a parent's written request to review and inspect them is pending. IDEA requires parental notification when a school district no longer needs a record "to provide educational services to the child." Parents may request destruction of unneeded information.

Guideline V

Require written, informed consent from the parent and, when appropriate, the student, to release medical and psychiatric diagnoses to other school personnel.

There are few circumstances when it is necessary to disclose a student's medical diagnosis. An emerging practice in schools is not to reveal any medical or psychiatric diagnoses to non-health professionals within the school without specific parental or student consent. While the medical or psychiatric diagnosis is not disclosed without consent, relevant health information necessary for educational planning and student safety can be shared among school personnel who serve the student. Functional health terminology is used rather than the diagnosis. If the school health professional determines that release of a diagnosis is relevant to the provision of appropriate health or educational services in school, having clear, easily understood confidentiality policies and informed consent procedures will help allay parents' concerns about giving consent. In turn, timely response from parents assures adequate continuity of care for students.

Informed Consent

The Youth Law Center identified 10 components that a consent form for release of confidential information regarding children and youth should include:[56]

1. Name of the person who is the subject of the information.

2. Name of the person, program, and agency releasing the information.

3. Name of the person, program, and agency with whom the information will be shared.

4. Reasons for sharing the information.

5. Kind of information that will be shared.

6. Signature of the person who is the subject of the information or, if a minor, the parent or legal guardian.

7. Date the release is signed.

8. A statement that the release can be revoked at any time by the subject of the information, or if the subject is a minor, the parent or legal guardian.

9. An expiration date or an event (such as the end of the school year, a statutory review date, or termination of assistance) that will terminate the release.

10. A statement that the signer has a right to a copy of the release.

Guideline VI

Limit the disclosure of confidential health information within the school to information necessary to benefit students' health or education.

A fundamental principle of FERPA is that student information is shared within the school on the basis of "legitimate educational interest" or "need to know."[4, 50, 57] Information "of interest" to a teacher or staff member might not be "necessary" to the provision of appropriate care or a student's success in school. The only information that should be shared is information that will directly benefit the student.

Functional Health Information

It is a clear violation of a student's privacy to have his or her name and diagnosis circulated on a "health problems list" to all teachers.[18-20, 34] If a student requires special assistance, the school health professional should contact individual teachers or administrators about the functional implications of the medical condition within the classroom and during other school activities, and provide written procedures necessary for health interventions, and emergency plans.[1]

The functional implication of a medical or psychiatric condition is what is most important to share with those having "legitimate educational interest." The National Task Force and others[20, 21, 58] recommend that school health professionals describe the functional strengths, limitations, and needs of the student when talking with educators and others working with the student. For example, nurses can share information about "fatigue" or "risk for activity intolerance" as defined by the North American Nursing Diagnosis Association,[58] enabling teachers and school staff to make appropriate accommodations in the classroom and during extracurricular activities without revealing the underlying diagnosis, which could be HIV infection, cystic fibrosis, or a myriad of other physical or psychological conditions.

Right to Know

"Need to know" should not be confused with "right to know." "Right to know" refers to citizens' rights to attend public meetings and obtain public records. These rights are protected by Freedom of Information Acts, or sunshine laws. Personnel files, medical records, and education records are NOT considered "public" records under these laws.[20, 59]

Guideline VII

Establish policies and standard procedures for requesting needed health information from outside sources and for releasing confidential health information, with parental consent, to outside agencies and individuals.

School health professionals may disclose confidential student health information to outside agencies that provide educational services to students on behalf of the district, e.g., a special education service or a city health department that provides school health services, only pursuant to a written contract or agreement with the school district. In this contract, the agency or organization acknowledges that it is fully bound by federal and state confidentiality laws and regulations as well as district policies. Such agreements should state how confidential information will be shared, with consent, unless otherwise allowed or required by law. The contract should also require the agency or organization to contest judicial initiatives to obtain confidential health information about a student, except as otherwise permitted by law.[5, 8, 60-63]

Occasionally, a school health professional needs advice or a professional opinion from a health care provider outside the school. Consultation about a particular student without parental consent is acceptable as long as the identity of the student and family is protected. Release of the name, address, birth date, or any other personal information about the student should not be necessary to fulfill the purpose of the consultation.[1] However, when information about a particular individual is required for planning purposes from other outside health care providers, hospitals, clinics, psychiatrists, or psychologists, it can only be obtained with informed consent of the parents, legal guardian, or the student (depending on age). With consent, the requested information will be sent to the school.

Without additional guidance, however, schools might receive unrequested or inappropriate information with little value for educational planning purposes. For this reason, all confidential health information should be sent only to an appropriate school health professional, even if requested for educational planning purposes. Health professionals should return unrequested information to the sender or shred it; it should NOT become part of the student's record. When unrequested information is sent, it is good practice to notify the student's parents.[1] If there is no school health professional in the district, there should be a written policy identifying, by title, the person to whom this type of information should be sent.

To limit the transfer of unnecessary information, school districts should send an individual cover letter explaining why specific information about the student is needed along with a signed parent consent form. The letter should also indicate the status of the record once it becomes part of the student's school health records (Figure 2-1). The ideal response to a school's request for health information is either a summary or selected excerpts from medical records that include the relevant physical, emotional, or psychological data needed to promote learning or provide appropriate related services, not the entire record.

School-based and School-linked Health Centers

The number of school-based and school-linked health centers has grown steadily in the last several years. In almost all cases, school-based and school-linked health centers are legally separate from the school system and are operated by independent contractors, therefore the center is an "outside agency."[8, 61, 62, 64] Parents must provide consent for their children to use the center's services and to bill the parents' insurance carrier. Some centers offer parents a "blanket" consent although this option might not be considered "informed" consent from a legal or ethical perspective. On a "checklist" consent, parents may exclude consent for some services such as reproductive health care. The consent form should also describe the types of health information that can be shared between the school health office and the center. In the rare case where the health center is actually operated by the school system, the confidentiality protections might differ, because FERPA and state education laws apply. Appendix D contains a model interagency agreement between a district and a school-based or school-linked health center.

Guideline VIII

Provide regular, periodic training for all new school staff, contracted service providers, substitute teachers, and school volunteers concerning the district's policies and procedures for protecting confidentiality.

Individuals with varied professional training work in schools, and the principles that guide their work often differ significantly. For health professionals, standards of practice regarding privacy and confidentiality are critical issues and considerable time is devoted to them in their professional preparation and training. On the other hand, the training and professional preparation of teachers, administrators, and other school staff might involve little discussion of student privacy and confidentiality.[1, 20, 21, 35] Paraprofessionals and community volunteers frequently receive no instruction in these concepts.

Such inconsistencies in training can lead to inappropriate disclosure or unnecessary withholding of information that results in physical, psychological, economic, or social harm to the individual and his or her family. In the case of poorly understood or socially charged situations such as adolescent pregnancy, HIV infection, or mental illness, affected individuals might experience recrimination, abandonment, or punishment.

Just as all teachers, other school staff, contractors, and volunteers should receive training about how to respond in health-related emergencies such as seizures, injuries involving the head and neck, bleeding, and asthma attacks, these same individuals should receive adequate information and regular, periodic training from their school districts on protecting confidentiality. Training should include a review of relevant federal and state laws, district policies and the disciplinary measures and sanctions for violating school confidentiality policy (Figure 2-2). In the event a licensed health professional violates confidentiality, the state regulatory board or other professional disciplinary authority should be notified. Finally, all school volunteers should sign an agreement to maintain the confidentiality of any student information they might learn while volunteering in school (Figure 2-3).

Figure 2-1
Sample Cover Letter to Accompany Parental Consent Form

May 20, 2000

John Smith, M.D.
Director of Pediatric Oncology
Pleasant Valley Hospital

Dear Dr. Smith:

Enclosed please find a signed consent form from the parents of **Susan L. Green** to release information about Susie to the school. According to the federal Individuals with Disabilities Education Act, Susie is eligible for special education services under the "Other Health Impaired" category. We are convening a team meeting in two weeks to plan an individualized education program (IEP) for her. The planning team includes the principal, her teacher, her occupational therapist, her parent(s) and me. The team will use the information you provide, along with data from our school records, to plan her academic program and to provide needed health services.

We need to know about her diagnoses, treatments, current health status, medications, and the monitoring she will need in school. In addition, please describe the current functional abilities and limitations she might have in the classroom or other school activities, as well as areas in which she might need support or program modification.

We prefer that you provide this information in a letter rather than as a full medical record. If you send copies of medical records, hospital records, or discharge summaries, please understand that per federal law, this material will become part of the school record. Our school district's policies restrict direct access to these records to authorized health care professionals and her parents although some of this information may be shared with other members of the IEP team or other teachers. Our practice is not to share a student's medical diagnosis without the specific consent of the parent. In addition, once a part of the school health record, the material you send will not be re-released without parental consent.

If you have questions about these polices or need additional information in regard to this request, please call me at 330/678-1603 x 129.

Sincerely,

Karen Washington, RN
Nursing Supervisor

Figure 2-2
School Staff Confidentiality Statement
Student Health Information

In the course of my employment or association with the school district, I understand that printed, electronic, and oral communications concerning ALL student health information are confidential. Such information can be accessed directly only by certain designated individuals and only for legitimate health purposes. Any keys to any files and any computer password assigned to me for which I am responsible will be kept confidential. Release of any student health information in printed, verbal, electronic, or any other form by unauthorized personnel is a major violation of school district standards for school employees and contracted service providers.

I have reviewed the school district's policies regarding confidentiality of student health information. I understand that improper release of student health information is cause for disciplinary action and can result in termination of employment and in some cases, civil liability.

If I have any questions concerning the confidentiality of student health information, I will consult my immediate supervisor or the school principal.

I have read, understand, and accept the above statements.

Signature of School Staff Member   Date

Note. Adapted from Guidelines for Policy and Practice: Confidentiality of Student Information., 1996, Connecticut Committee on Confidentiality of Student Information, Middletown, Conn: Connecticut State Dept. of Education. used with permission of Connecticut State Dept. of Education.

Figure 2-3
**School District Volunteer
Agreement Not to Disclose
Confidential Student Information**

Please print.

| Last Name | First Name | Middle Initial | Telephone |

Address

   I understand that ALL student information to which I have access as a school volunteer is confidential. Such information might include health information in written, oral, or electronic form. I agree not to discuss any confidential information, including but not limited to any descriptions of situations as well as names of students. I also understand that even when I am no longer a volunteer for the school district, confidential information I have learned as a volunteer must continue to be kept confidential.

   I understand that any breach of the confidentiality of student information will result in my immediate termination as a volunteer in the school district and that I may be subject to civil liability in some cases.

   Other provisions (May vary from school district to school district)

   My signature indicates that I promise to share confidential student health information only with authorized school health professionals. My signature on this form indicates that I understand and agree to comply with the conditions stated in the school district policies provided to me and on this form.

| Volunteer's signature | Date |

Note: Modified from the Iowa Dept. of Human Services Volunteer Registration Form.

REFERENCES

1) Connecticut Committee on Confidentiality of Student Health Information (1996). Draft *Guidelines for policy and practice: Confidentiality of student information.* Middletown, CT: Connecticut State Department of Education.

2) Individuals with Disabilities Education Act, 20 U.S.C.A. 1400 et seq., particularly regulations at 34 C.F.R. 300.560-577 IDEA) Formerly called the Education of All Handicapped Children Act, or EHA.

3) Rehabilitation Act of 1973, Section 504; 29 U.S.C.A. 793, regulations at 34 C.F.R. 104.

4) Cheung, O., Clements, B., & Pechman, E. (1997). *Protecting the privacy of student records: Guidelines for education agencies.* Council of Chief State School Officers, prepared for the National Forum on Education Statistics, under the National Center for Education Statistics, U.S. Department of Education, Washington, D.C.

5) Committee on Maintaining Privacy and Security in Health Care Applications of the National Information Infrastructure. (1997). *For the record: Protecting electronic health information.* Washington, DC: National Academy Press.

6) National Education Association. (1991). *NEA handbook, 1991-92.* Washington, DC: National Education Association.

7) Ford, C.A, Millstein, S.G., Halpern-Felsher, B.L., & Irwin, C.E. (1997). Influence of physician confidentiality assurances on adolescents' willingness to disclose information and seek future health care. *Journal of American Medical Association,* 278 (12):1029-1034. Cited in Digests. (1998) *Family Planning Perspectives,* 301):52.

8) Loxterman, J. (1997). Adolescent access to confidential health services. *Issues at a Glance.* Washington, DC: Advocates for Youth.

9) American Occupational Therapy Association. (1994). Guidelines to the Occupational Therapy Code of Ethics. *American Journal of Occupational Therapy,* 52 10):881-884.

10) American Speech-Language-Hearing Association. (1995). Code of Ethics in *Membership*

and certification handbook. Rockville, MD: American Speech-Language-Hearing Association.

11) National Association of School Nurses. (1990). *Code of ethics.* Scarborough, ME: National Association of School Nurses.

12) Proctor, S.T., Lordi, S.L., & Zaiger, D.S. (1993). *School nursing practice: Roles and standards.* Scarborough, ME: National Association of School Nurses.

13) Holder, A.R. (1988). Disclosure and consent: Problems in pediatrics. *Law, Medicine & Health Care,* 16 (3-4).

14) Husted, G.L., & Husted, J.H. (1995). *Ethical decision making in nursing* (2nd ed.). St. Louis, MO: Mosby.

15) Rushton, C. Address to National Task Force on Confidential Student Health Information. Washington, D.C., March 1996.

16) Arnold v. Board of Education of Escambia County, Alabama, 754 F.Supp. 853 S.D. Ala. (1990).

17) Fischer, L., & Sorenson, G.P. (1996). *School law for counselors, psychologists, and social workers* 3rd Ed.). White Plains, NY: Longman.

18) Schwab, N. (1988). Liability issues in school nursing. *School Nurse,* 4 (1): 17-21.

19) Schwab, N.C., & Gelfman, M.H.B. (1991). School health records: Nursing practice and the law. *School Nurse,* 7: 26-34.

20) Schwab, N., & Gelfman, M.J. (Eds.). in press) *Legal issues in school health services: A reference for school nurses, administrators and attorneys.* North Branch, MN: Sunrise River Press.

21) Schwab, N., Panettieri, M.J., & Bergren, M. (1998). *Guidelines for school nursing documentation: Standards, issues and models* (2nd ed.). Scarborough, ME: National Association of School Nurses.

22) Sibner, unpublished letter from LeRoy Rooker, Family Policy Compliance Office, U.S. Department of Education, March 14, 1994.

23) Armijo vs. Wagon Mound Public Schools, 159F3d 1253 10th Cir. (1998).

24) Tarasoff v. Regents of the University of California, 551 P.2d 334 (Cal. 1976).

25) Swartz, M. (1990). Is there a Duty to Warn? *Human Rights,* 17 (1): 40.

26) Legal Action Center of the City of New York. (1996). *Legal issues for school based programs.* New York, NY: Author.

27) American Federation of Teachers. (1997). *The medically fragile child in the school setting.* Washington, DC: American Federation of Teachers.

28) Family Educational Rights and Privacy Act, 20 U.S.C.A. 1232g, regulations at 34 C.F.R. Part 99 FERPA, sometimes called the Buckley Amendment.

29) Billings, J., Pearson, J., Carthum, H., & Maire, J. (1995). *Guidelines for handling health care information in school records.* Olympia, WA: Superintendent of Public Instruction.

30) Massachusetts Department of Education. 1995). *Student records: Questions, answers, and guidelines.* Malden, MA: Massachusetts Department of Education.

31) Goodman, I.F., & Sheetz, A.H. Eds. (1995). *The comprehensive school health manual.* Boston: Massachusetts Department of Public Health.

32) Maryland Department of Education. (1992). *Confidentiality guidelines for student education records and communications.* Baltimore, MD: Maryland Department of Education.

33) Oregon Department of Education. (1996). Health records/medical records/confidentiality. In *Health services for the school community,* pp. 15-19. Salem, OR: Oregon Department of Education.

34) Gelfman, M., & Schwab, N. (1991). School health services and education records: Conflicts in the law. *Education Law Reports,* 64:319-338.

35) Siegler, G.E. (1996). What should be the scope of privacy protections for student health records? A look at Massachusetts and federal law. *Journal of Law and Education,* 25 (2): 237- 269.

36) Medaris, M.L., Campbell, E., & James, B. (1997). Sharing information: *A guide to the Family Educational Rights and Privacy Act and participation in juvenile justice programs.* Washington, DC: U.S. Department of Justice Office of Juvenile Justice and Delinquency Prevention and U.S. Department of Education Family Policy Compliance Office.

37) Protection of Pupil Rights Amendment, 20 U.S.C.A. 1232h sometimes called the Hatch Amendment.

38) English, A., Matthews, M., Extavour, K., Palamountain, C., & Yang, J. (1995). *State minor consent statutes: A summary.* Cincinnati, OH: Center for Continuing Education in Adolescent Health, Division of Adolescent Medicine, Children's Hospital Medical Center.

39) Holder, A.R. (1985). *Legal issues in pediatrics and adolescent medicine* (2nd ed.). New Haven, CT: Yale University Press.

40) Holder, A.R. (1987). Minors' rights to consent to medical care. *Journal of the American Medical Association,* 257 (24): 3400-3402.

41) Morrissey, J.M. (1997). *Rights and responsibilities of young people in New York.* Albany, NY: New York State Bar Association.

42) Reed, S. (1988). Children with AIDS: How schools are handling this crisis. Kappan Special Report. *Phi Delta Kappan,* 69 (5): K1-K12.

43) Reed, S. (1986) AIDS in the schools: A special report. *Phi Delta Kappan,* 67 (7), 494-498.

44) Ray v. School District of DeSoto County, 666 F.Supp. 1524 M.D.Fla. (1987).

45) *Board of Education of the City of Plainfield v. Cooperman,* 507 A.2d 253 N.J.Super.A.D. (1986); 523 A.2d 655 N.J. (1987).

46) *Child v. Spillane,* 875 F.2d 314, EHLR Dec. 441:101 4th Cir. (1989).

47) *District 27 Community School Board v. Board of Education of the City of New York,* 130 Misc.2d 398, 502 N.Y.S.2d 325, EHLR Dec. 557:241 Sup.Ct. NY (1986).

48) Bogden, J.F., Fraser, K., Vega-Matos, C., & Ascroft, J. (1996). *Someone at school has AIDS: A complete guide to education policies concerning HIV information,* Alexandria, VA: National Association of State Boards of Education.

49) National Parent Teachers Association. (1997). *Parent involvement standards.* Chicago: National PTA.

50) *Guidelines for the Collection, Maintenance & Dissemination of Pupil Records: Report of a*

Conference on the Ethical & Legal Aspects of School Record Keeping Sterling Forest, NY, (May 25-28, 1969). (1970). New York: Russell Sage Foundation.

51) Johnson, T.P. (1993). Managing student records: The courts and the Family Educational Rights and Privacy Act of 1974. *Education Law Reports,* 79: 319 Feb. 11, 1993.

52) U.S. Department of Education. (1995). *Student records policies and procedures for Alpha School District.* Washington, DC: Author.

53) Schluessler v. Independent School District No. 200, 1989 Minnesota Case Reports 652, Dakota County Court.

54) Hedberg, S.M. (1997). A comparative analysis of PC-based school health software. *Journal of School Nursing,* 13 (1): 30-38.

55) Hedberg, S.M. (1997). Administrative student information management software AS/IMS) for school nurse record keeping and reporting. *Journal of School Nursing,* 13 (2): 40-48.

56) Soler, M.I., Shotton, A.C., & Bell, J.R. (1993). *Glass walls: Confidentiality provisions and interagency collaboration.* San Francisco, CA: Youth Law Center.

57) Zirkel, P. (1997). Disclosure of student records: A comprehensive overview. *The Special Educator,* 12 (16): 1,4.

58) North American Nursing Diagnosis Association. (1997-98). *Nursing diagnosis: Definitions and classifications.* Philadelphia: Author.

59) Rosenfeld, S.J., Gelfman, M.H.B., & Bluth, L.F. (1997). *Education Records: A Manual.* Hollywood, FL: EDLAW, Inc.

60) Goslin, L.O., Tarek-Brezina, J., Powers, M., Kozloff, R., Faden, R., & Steinauer, D. (1993). Privacy and security of personal information in a new health care system. *Journal of the American Medical Association,* 270 (20): 2487-2493.

61) Joining Forces, American Public Welfare Association, Center for Law and Social Policy, Council of Chief State School Officers & Education Commission of the States. (1992). *Confidentiality and collaboration: Information sharing in interagency efforts.* Denver, CO: Education Commission of the States.

62) Loxterman, J., & English, A., Ed. (1996). *A guide to school-based and school-linked health centers,* Vol. V: Introduction to legal issues. Washington, DC: Advocates for Youth.

63) Soler, M.I., Shotton, A.C., & Bell, J.R. (1995). *Model form for consent to exchange confidential information among the members of an interagency collaborative.* San Francisco, CA: Youth Law Center.

64) Nader, P.R. (Ed.) (1993). *School health: Policy and practice.* Elk Grove Village, IL: American Academy of Pediatrics.

APPENDIX A

DEFINITIONS

Agency/Agencies - Local public school systems, regional, and state public education facilities; public and private family service organizations; private schools and facilities providing special education and early intervention services; and state departments of education and other state departments providing services to children.[1]

Aides - see **Paraprofessional**.

Client - In education settings, the student; in health care settings, the patient; the parent or guardian when the student is a minor. In early childhood programs, the infant or toddler and family.[1]

Common and Case Law - Legal principles developed from court decisions. Decisions are usually binding only for closely similar facts in the same jurisdiction, but sometimes have advisory force in other jurisdictions or in analogous circumstances.

Confidential Information - Information, that if disclosed by someone other than the individual, would likely constitute an invasion of personal privacy.[1] The individual providing information controls that information, and, with few exceptions, must consent before anyone else may release the information. All school records with personally identifiable information about a student are confidential under FERPA. Medical records with personally identifiable information are confidential under federal and state laws.

Disclosure - To permit access to or the release, transfer, or other communication of personally identifiable information contained in education records to any party, by any means, including oral, written, or electronic. (34 CFR 99.3)

Education Records - Records that are 1) directly related to a student and 2) maintained by, or on behalf of, schools. "Records" includes information recorded in any way, including, but not limited to, handwriting, print, computer media, video or audio tape, film, microfilm, and microfiche. (34 CFR 99.3)

Family - The immediate household members with whom a child lives, and the "extended family," relatives and others, who assist in care and support of the child. In many cases, the family defines itself.

Health Care Services - Any service or procedure provided by a health care provider to diagnose, treat, maintain, or improve a person's physical or emotional status; or that affects the structure or any function of the body; or that promotes healthy lifestyles. Services provided in school pursuant to a special education Individualized Education Program (IEP) or a Section 504 accommodation plan are usually called school health services, related services, or support services.

Health Care Provider - A licensed health professional. Each state defines by licensing requirements who is considered a health care provider in that state.

Health Status -The physical, developmental, social, and mental health condition of an individual.[1]

Individualized Education Program (IEP) - A written plan required for all students receiving special education and related services. The IEP is developed by a team of school professionals, in a meeting with the student's parent(s) (34 CFR 300.340 - 300.350).

Individualized Health Program (IHP) - A written plan, developed by a school nurse or by a school health team, to determine desired student outcomes and appropriate health services for a student who requires nursing services or other health-related support in school.

Licensure - Procedure established under state law that sets standards for permitting professional practice such as for physicians, nurses, psychologists, social workers, and teachers. See also Professional Certification.

Local School District - As designated under state law, the area served by a public school system. Depending on state law, a local school district might include one or more schools, elementary and/or secondary schools, or both; or one or more towns or municipalities. A local school district is usually governed by a board of education.

Mental Health Professionals - Individuals licensed or certified to attend to emotional and social health needs. These include psychiatrists, psychologists, and social workers.

Paraprofessionals - Usually non-licensed and non-certified personnel. In the school they work under the direct supervision of a teacher, school nurse, or other school health professional.

Parent - A biological parent, a guardian legally responsible for a minor, or an adult acting as a parent (34 CFR 300.13, including note).

Patient - A person consulting or being treated by a health care provider.

Personnel - Individuals employed by the school district; sometimes referred to as "school staff."

Privacy, right of - An individual's right to withhold personal information from others.

Professional Certification - Procedures established by state law that define the requirements for a professional credential; usually required for employment as a teacher or health care provider in any public school. A certificate may be permanent or issued for a specific term, such as 5 or 10 years. See also **Licensure**.

Pupil Services Professionals - Health, mental health, and education professionals employed by the school and provide services that support the learning process. Such staff includes, but is not limited to school nurses, counselors, school psychologists, social workers, occupational and physical therapists, and speech pathologists. Not all pupil services professionals are licensed health providers.

Medical Records - Documentation of consultation or treatment by a health care provider, usually defined and protected under state law.

School-Based, School-Linked Health Centers - A professionally staffed health center on or near school grounds established to provide a comprehensive range of services for students and their families. In most cases the centers are legally separate from the school system.

School Administrator - A state-certified school superintendent, principal, or other supervisory school official.

School Medical Advisor - A physician employed by a school district as a consultant. Not all states or school districts require such a consultant.

School Nurse - A licensed, professional registered nurse (RN) whose practice focuses on health promotion and the health care needs of students in the school community. State nurse practice laws define licensure requirements for nurses. State law may define specific qualifications for school nurses, eg, some states require certification of school nurses under teacher certification laws. School nurses can be directly employed by the school district or by public health or other agencies such as school-based or school-linked health centers.

Student - Any individual who is or has been in attendance at an educational agency or institution and regarding whom the agency or institution maintains education records. Any infant or toddler who is or has been in attendance at an early intervention program that is under the auspices of a designated state agency (34 CFR 99.3).[1]

Student Information - Includes, but is not limited to, written, electronic and oral communication concerning a student's academic performance; health and developmental history; disciplinary history; counseling data; mental health history; a variety of testing and evaluation data; disability status; records from outside health care providers or agencies; and family information, including but not limited to biographic, sociodemographic, insurance, financial, and health data (34 CFR 99.3).[1]

Teacher - A person who meets or is expected to meet the state requirements for licensure or certification to instruct students in public elementary or secondary schools.

APPENDIX B

List of National Reviewers

Sue Abderholden
PACER Center

Karlene Abrams
UNCF HOPE Program

Scott G. Allen
American Academy of Pediatrics

Olga Acosta, PhD
Center for School Mental Health Assistance

Dara Bass
Kentucky School Boards Association

Nancy Birchmeier, BSN, CSN, RN
National Association of School Nurses

Beverly Bradley, PhD, RN
University of California, San Diego

Ellen Campbell
U.S. Dept. of Education

Carol Costante, MA, RN, CSN, FNASN
National Association of School Nurses

Victoria Duran
National Parent Teacher Association

Mary Gannon
Iowa Association of School Boards

Robert Gellman
Privacy and Information Policy Consultant

Paul R. Getto
Kansas Association of School Boards

Gabriella Hayes
National Parent Teacher Association

Janis Hootman, PhD, BSN, RN
Multnomah (Wash.) Education Services District

Dixie Snow Huefner
University of Utah

Shirley Igo
National Parent Teacher Association

Judith B. Igoe, MS, RN, FAAN
University of Colorado

Carol J. Iverson, MSN, RN, CSN
Nebraska Dept. of Health and Human Services

Leslie Jackson, MEd, OT
American Occupational Therapy Association, Inc.

Lauren B. Kingsbery, Esq.
Colorado Association of School Boards

Sandy Landry, MEd, RN, PNP
Orange County (Calif.) Dept. of Education

Doris Luckenbill, MS, CRNP, RN
National Association of School Nurses

Judith A. Maire, MN, RN
Olympia (Wash.) Public Schools

Naomi Marsh, MEd
New York State Education Dept.

Jonathan McIntire, PhD
Council of Administrators of Special Education, Inc.

Sue McKee, RN, CSN
Lindbergh (Mo.) School District

Judy Mountjoy
National Parent Teacher Association

Vincent A. Mustaro
Connecticut Association of Boards of Education, Inc.

Maribeth Oakes
National Parent Teacher Association

Carol Paladino, RN, BA, CSN
National Association of School Nurses

Mary Jane K. Rappaport, PhD, PT
University of Colorado Health Sciences Center

Mary Ann Roll
National Parent Teacher Association

S. James Rosenfeld, Esq.
EDLAW, Inc.

Cynthia Rushton, DDSc, FAAN
Johns Hopkins University

Diane S. Scalise, MS, RN
School Board of Broward County (Fla.)

Julie M. Slavens, Esq.
Indiana School Boards Association

Yvonne Swinth, PhD, OTR/L
School of Occupational Therapy & Physical Therapy

Gwen Tucker
National Parent Teacher Association

Jane Tustin, MSN, CSN, RN
National Association of School Nurses

Genie Wessel, MS, RN
University of Maryland School of Nursing/MCH

Michael Wessely
National School Boards Association

Gordon Wrobel
National Association of School Psychologists

Wayne A. Yankus, MD
American Academy of Pediatrics

APPENDIX C

Model Notification of Rights Under FERPA for Elementary And Secondary Institutions

The Family Educational Rights and Privacy Act (FERPA) affords parents and students older than 18 years of age ("eligible students") certain rights with respect to the student's education records. They are:

(1) The right to inspect and review the student's education records within 45 days of the day the District receives a request for access.

Parents or eligible students should submit to the school principal [or appropriate school official] a written request that identifies the record(s) they wish to inspect. The principal will make arrangements for access and notify the parent or eligible student of the time and place where the records may be inspected.

(2) The right to request the amendment of the student's education records that the parent or eligible student believes are inaccurate or misleading.

Parents or eligible students may ask Alpha School District to amend a record they believe is inaccurate or misleading. They should write the school principal, clearly identify the part of the record they want changed, and specify why it is inaccurate or misleading.

If the District decides not to amend the record as requested by the parent or eligible student, the District will notify the parent or eligible student of the decision and advise them of their right to a hearing regarding the request for amendment. Additional information regarding the hearing procedures will be provided to the parent or eligible student when notified of the right to a hearing.

(3) The right to consent to disclosures of personally identifiable information contained in the student's education records, except to the extent that FERPA authorizes disclosure without consent.

One exception that permits disclosure without consent is disclosure to school officials with legitimate educational interests. A school official is a person employed by the District as an administrator, supervisor, instructor, or support staff member (including health or medical staff and law enforcement unit personnel); a person serving on the School Board; a person or company with whom the District has contracted to perform a special task (such as an attorney, auditor, medical consultant, or therapist); or a parent or student serving on an official committee, such as a disciplinary or grievance committee, or assisting another school official in performing his or her tasks.

A school official has a legitimate educational interest if the official needs to review an education record in order to fulfill his or her professional responsibility.

[Optional] Upon request, the District discloses education records without consent to officials of another school district in which a student seeks or intends to enroll. [NOTE: FERPA requires a school district to make a reasonable attempt to notify the student of the records request unless it states in its annual notification that it intends to forward records on request.]

(4) The right to file a complaint with the U.S. Department of Education concerning alleged failures by the District to comply with the requirements of FERPA. The name and address of the Office that administers FERPA:

Family Policy Compliance Office
U.S. Dept. of Education
600 Independence Ave., SW
Washington, DC 20202-4605

APPENDIX D

Model Interagency Agreement

This Agreement made and entered into as of the date set forth below, by and between [List Agencies Here]

WITNESSETH:

WHEREAS, all parties are committed to providing appropriate programs and services to promote children's health and success in school and intervene with children at risk for health or behavioral problems; and

WHEREAS, the parties to this agreement desire a maximum degree of long range cooperation and administrative planning to provide for the health and safety of the community and its children; and

WHEREAS, all parties are committed to improving services to children in schools and the community through sharing information, eliminating duplication of services, and coordinating efforts; and

WHEREAS, all parties mutually agree that sharing resources, where feasible, and in particular, training efforts, may result in improved coordination; and

WHEREAS, it is the understanding of all parties that certain roles in serving children and youth are required by law, and that these laws serve as the foundation for defining the role and responsibility of each participating agency; and

WHEREAS, all parties mutually agree that all obligations stated or implied in this agreement shall be interpreted in light of, and consistent with, governing State and Federal laws;

NOW, THEREFORE, in consideration of the following agreements, the parties do hereby covenant and agree to do the following:

EACH OF THE PARTIES AGREES TO:

1. Promote a coordinated effort among agencies and staff to achieve maximum health and academic success of school-aged children and youth.

2. Participate in interagency planning meetings, as appropriate.

3. Assign staff, as appropriate, to participate in planning individualized education or health plans, re-entry into school of children returning from illness or treatment programs, other information-sharing activities to assess and develop plans for medically-fragile, special education, at-risk youth, or students in need of health or psychosocial health services.

4. Jointly plan and provide information and access to training opportunities when feasible.

5. Develop internal policies and cooperative procedures, as needed, to implement this agreement to the maximum extent possible.

6. Comply with relevant State and Federal law and other applicable school district policies and administrative procedures that relate to records use, security, dissemination, and retention or destruction.

THE COLLABORATING AGENCY AGREES TO:

1. Notify the Health Services Coordinator, or designee, of the name and address of any student found to require an adaptive program or special health services in school. Notification shall include the specific functional capabilities or limitations for which collaborative planning and services will be necessary.

2. Suggest strategies and techniques to maximize the student's health, safety, and academic progress in school.

3. Upon request by the school district, share appropriate information with the Health Services Coordinator or his or her designee regarding students within the educational system for purposes of assessment, placement, or evaluation.

4. Consider the assignment of staff necessary to promote the goals of this agreement, particularly information sharing between the agencies involved.

5. Develop, in cooperation with School, the family, and collaborating service providers, a written plan to determine the procedures to take when a child is identified as being in a medical or psychiatric crisis.

6. Develop appropriate internal written policies to ensure that confidential health record information is disseminated only to appropriate personnel.

THE SCHOOL HEALTH SERVICES OFFICE AGREES TO:

1. Contact the collaborating service provider immediately upon learning of the health and safety status needs of the student in school.

2. Share dispositional, placement, and case management information with other agencies as appropriate for purposes of assessment, placement, and enhanced success in school.

3. Develop, in cooperation with School, the family, and collaborating service providers, a written plan to determine the procedures to take when a child requires modifications of the individualized health or education plan.

4. Develop appropriate internal written policies to ensure that confidential health information is disseminated only to appropriate and duly authorized personnel.

5. Share information on student achievement and program modifications implemented in schools to reduce risk and promote school success for the purpose of assessment and treatment.

6. Develop, in cooperation with School, the family, and local service providers, a written plan to determine the procedures to take when a child is identified as being in a medical or psychiatric crisis.

THE SCHOOL DISTRICT ADMINISTRATION AGREES TO:

1. Provide notice to the Board of Education, immediately upon the initiation of planning efforts with private nonprofit entities or governmental entities, including agencies part of this Agreement, that could result in the creation, relocation, or expansion of health services or programs that might affect the school district.

2. Develop recommendations for policies that support health and psychosocial health services in schools in cooperation with members of the faculty, school health professionals, family representatives, and collaborating service providers. Such recommendations should also specify appropriate sanctions if these policies and administrative procedures are violated.

3. Develop clearly written administrative procedures that ensure that confidential health information is disseminated only to appropriate personnel.

THE BUILDING PRINCIPAL AGREES TO:

1. Notify the child's teachers of his or her support for collaborative health planning on behalf of the student.

2. Designate the collaborating teacher, if more than one is involved, responsible for serving on the student's IEP planning team.

3. Participate as a member of the child's IEP planning team, as appropriate.

4. Inform teachers and other support staff of the name of the authorized contact person(s) responsible for receiving confidential health information.

5. Implement administrative procedures to ensure that confidential health information is disseminated only to appropriate school personnel.

6. Notify the Superintendent, or designee, of the name of any employee of the school district or volunteer who violates the district's policies and

administrative procedures for protecting the privacy and confidentiality of students' health information.

ADMINISTRATIVE

TERM OF AGREEMENT:

This agreement shall be in effect as of the date the agreement is signed by all the initiating parties and shall renew automatically unless otherwise modified. Any party signatory to this agreement may terminate participation upon thirty days notice to all other signed parties to the agreement.

AGENCY REPRESENTATIVES:

The parties will develop procedures for ongoing meetings and will at least annually review and, if necessary, recommend any changes.

MODIFICATION OF AGREEMENT:

Modification of this agreement shall be made only by consent of the majority of the initiating parties. Such shall be made with the same formalities as were followed in this agreement and shall include a written document setting forth the modifications, signed by all the consenting parties.

SIGNATURES OF PARTIES TO THIS AGREEMENT:

Upon signing this agreement, the original agreement and signature shall be filed with the Superintendent's office and placed in the public records of the district. A certified copy of the agreement and the signatures shall be provided to each signatory to the agreement.

OTHER INTERAGENCY AGREEMENTS:

All parties to this agreement acknowledge that this agreement does not preclude or preempt each of the

agencies individually entering into an agreement
with one or more parties to this agreement. Such
agreements shall not nullify the force and effect of
this agreement. This agreement does not remove any
other obligations imposed by law to share information
with other agencies.

Signed _____

Title _____

Date _____